Prostate Cancer Seed Therapy (Brachytherapy):

An Alternative to Surgery and Its Side Effects

Lonnie Boyd

ISBN:1723500267
ISBN-13:978-172350026 8

CONTENTS

	About This Book	i
1	The Prostate: Makes a Man a Man	1
2	Prostate Cancer Is not the good cancer	Pg 4
3	Smorgasboard of Possible Treatments	Pg 7
4	My Personal Prostate Journey Begins	Pg 12
5	Risk Factors For Prostate Cancer	Pg 21
6	Comparing Brachytherapy and Surgery	Pg 24
7	Radiation Oncology Consult	Pg 28

8	My Operation and Typical Results	Pg 35
9	The Aftermath	Pg 43
10	Additional Resources	Pg 47

About This Book

You can beat prostate cancer! And many men have found a way to do so without prostate removal surgery and its sometimes severe side effects! This book recommends "Seeds versus Scalpels", or brachytherapy versus prostate surgery.

I am a 13 year prostate cancer survivor. I chose not to have prostate removal and opted for radiation seed therapy or brachytherapy instead. As a result of my research at the time I decided that my recovery from the procedure and chances of avoiding severe side effects would be better with seeds instead of scalpels. In fact that is how my story played out.

 In this book I present a plain language explanation of some challenging and complex medical issues I faced, It is my hope that this discussion will help you as you face many of those same challenges. I am not a doctor, but I have been through the prostate wars and have lived to tell about it

The following chapters tell my story and share the research I performed in order to inform my decisions.

Some material in this book was previous;y

published in my earlier book <u>How To Avoid Prostate Surgery Side Effects.</u>

What This Book Is Not

This book does not attempt to be a highly complex explanation of the latest advances and controversies in cancer treatment. We will not go into, nor would it be possible to discuss, all the latest treatment fads and the ever changing opinions on them.

This book details my prostate cancer journey. I discuss the choices I made in overcoming fear and seeking the best and safest treatment. This book is no replacement for the individual medical attention you need. What worked for me might not work for you. And then again it might. Each man's cancer is different. Each man's life circumstances are different. Each man's tolerance for the trade off of side effects for possible cure is different

I believe it is essential for every man to work out his treatment choices with his medical team, his significant other and his God.

1.THE PROSTATE: TO SOME PEOPLE, IT MAKES A MAN A MAN

Overview of the Prostate

Let's look at some basic information about the prostate. Like I was, many men are ignorant about their prostate up to the point where things go haywire, affecting their bathroom habits or their sexual functioning.

The prostate is a small gland, in most men about the size of a walnut or golf ball. It is nestled so deep in a man's pelvis that a doctor will stick his finger up a man's rear end to feel it. The prostate plays key roles in both urination and ejaculation. Because of this the prostate can affect those things that we sometimes think make us a man;

sex and peeing standing up. Yes, intellectually I know those are not the things that make a man a man, but my emotions and ego sometimes say otherwise.

The ureter that carries urine from the bladder to the penis runs through the prostate. Because of this anatomy, prostate removal, whether open surgery or robotic surgery, requires the surgeon to cut the ureter and stitch it back together. One of the sphincters that turns urine flow on and off is removed when the prostate is removed, greatly increasing the chances of leakage.

The prostate also plays a leading role in male sexuality. Most of the ingredients of semen are produced by the prostate. When the prostate is removed, men will have a "dry" orgasm or even leak urine with their orgasm. Orgasms themselves are very different without the prostate. At orgasm, the prostate clutches and pumps out the semen it produced.

As another risk and complication, the nerves that control erections run along the outer edges of the prostate and are often damaged in surgery. There is a large market for "nerve sparing prostatectomy"' but it is not always possible to spare them. Much depends on the location of the cancer and the skill of the surgeon. 100 per cent of prostate surgery patients do not have erections for a period after the surgery and may not regain them.

2 PROSTATE CANCER IS NOT "THE GOOD CANCER"

Often well meaning friends, coworkers or even strangers will tell a man, "Thank goodness you don't have one of the BAD cancers." Or "If you have to have cancer, prostate cancer is not so bad. You are more likely to die with it than of it".

There is often some truth in platitudes. But this platitude can be deceptive and misleading. Some cases of prostate cancer do have a great survival rate, although the side effects of treatment can still be scary. But other cases of prostate cancer can be a nightmare for the patient and their family.

Prostate cancer is a killer. The American Cancer Society estimates that in 2017 there will be over 26,000 men die from prostate cancer, and about 161,000 new cases. In addition to those whom the cancer actually kills, the stress and side effects involved with prostate cancer contribute to the deaths of untold additional men each year.

Just hearing that the words "You have cancer", is a shock to most men. Finding out about the side effects of a potential cure will be even more of a gut check... .Surgical removal of the prostate can leave men impotent and leaking urine.

A Harvard University study published in 2009 (ABC News 12/15/2009) interviewed more than 4 million Swedish men and found that a diagnosis of prostate cancer increased the relative risks for fatal heart problems by 11 times and the suicide rate over 8 times in the week following their diagnosis.

The ABC article goes on to say that men who don't develop heart problems or commit suicide (most of us, thank God) commonly deal with depression in the months following diagnosis and treatment. Impotence and urinary incontinence can be very depressing. In addition men often must follow up surgery (or radiation) with hormone therapy. This treatment can also result in impotence and loss of desire for sex. These are hard consequences for the fragile male ego to face.

3 A SMORGASBORD OF POSSIBLE TREATMENTS

I read online that there were 4 treatments that seemed the most likely to be offered to me when I had my initial diagnosis of prostate cancer. The choices included surgery, radiation (either external or seeds), hormone therapy and cryotherapy. Each has several subsets, with more being added every year.   My initial research yielded the following:

Surgery

I read a lot of horror stories about diapers and impotence after surgery. There seemed to be a lot of surgery patients who were glad to no longer have cancer, but who were surprised and upset about the side effects they were experiencing.

Because the ureter runs through the prostate, it must be cut out along with the prostate, and the ends on both sides of the surgery stitched together again. This necessitates the use of a catheter for weeks after the operation. It has been estimated that ten percent of men never regain full urinary continence.

The situation around sexual functioning can be even more concerning. Some estimates indicated that up to 60 percent of men do not recover sexually. Even if a man does regains sexual functioning, it will never be the same. Most of the ejaculate is produced by the prostate gland, and at climax the prostate "clutches" to deliver the product, so to speak. A missing prostate means a very changed climax. Also, the nerves that help with erections run along each side of the prostate and are often damaged during surgery. And let us not even address the rumors of penile shrinkage.

A number of surgery patients in the chat groups pointed out, "Dead men don't have sex!" making the point that perhaps saving your life and losing your sex life was better than doing the opposite. I held out hope that there might be a better way.

Radiation

At the time I was diagnosed, there were two basic forms of radiation treatment offered. EBRT (External Beam Radiation Therapy) involved a number of treatments where a beam of radiation was targeted at a particular part of the body. Brachytherapy, or Seeds, came in two forms. LDR (Low Dose Radiation), involved the placing of a number of titanium pellets the size of a grain of rice and filled with a radioactive material permanently in the prostate. As the radiation was slowly released, the cancer cells were destroyed. In HDR (High Dose Radiation), a stronger source of radiation was temporarily placed in the prostate, then removed. Radiation, either external or seeds, seemed to have fewer side effects to begin with than surgery, but the side effects often worsened later. Additionally, not everyone qualified for either external or internal radiation depending on the extent and aggressiveness of their cancer.

Hormone Therapy

Hormone therapy, otherwise known as anti-androgen therapy, is used either alone or in combination with other therapies. Hormone therapy alone does not cure prostate cancer, instead it aims to slow its growth.

Androgens are the male hormones testosterone and DHT. They are known to "feed" prostate cancer. Reducing their production slows the growth of the cancer for a time. Androgens are primarily produced in the testicles, with a smaller amount produced in the adrenal glands.

The original androgen deprivation treatment was orchiectomy, or surgical removal of the testicles, otherwise known as castration. This is the least expensive option for hormone therapy, but most men do not choose it, both for psychological reasons and because it is so, so permanent.

The varied drug treatments are referred to as chemical castration. They can be used for a limited time or intermittently. Hormone therapy is often used in combination with surgery or radiation.

Common side effects include loss of libido, impotence, shrinkage of the sexual organs, fatigue and mental fog.

Cryotherapy

Cryotherapy involves sticking very cold probes into prostate and freezing the cancer cells to death. In 2005 it was a relatively new and little used treatment. It was reported to have about a 100 per cent chance of impotence. At my age I was not ready for that.

The treatment choices become even more complex in cases of advanced prostate cancer, but I did not have to deal with that at that time, I hoped. Those were the cases where it was known that the cancer had already spread outside the prostate.

4 MY PERSONAL PROSTATE JOURNEY BEGINS

I began my treatment at the University of Kansas Hospital in Kansas City Kansas, otherwise referred to as KU Medical Center This was not on the basis of research, but rather because my primary care doctor practiced there.

KU Cancer Center has been a National Cancer Centers (NCC) Center of Excellence since 2012. They were not yet there in 2005 when my treatment began. Note: For the most part I have been very pleased with the care I received at KU Hospital. I am not qualified to give a thorough analysis their services, but you may consider this a glowing endorsement from one long time patient.

My prostate journey began when my primary care doctor referred me to a Urologist. She was concerned about some blood test results from my annual checkup. The blood test that concerned her was a PSA test. I didn't know what that meant.

Definition of PSA

I now know that PSA stands for Prostate Specific Antigen. This is a protein produced in the prostate which becomes an ingredient in a man's semen. One source I read stated that PSA is what makes semen sticky. While most of the PSA is used in semen production, a certain amount of it ends up in the bloodstream. This is what the PSA blood test measures.

Prostate cancer cells also produce PSA, but all of the PSA they produce ends up in the blood raising the PSA blood level. A high PSA blood level is not definitive for cancer, but it is a sign that more examination may be needed. The PSA level can also be raised by the natural enlargement of the prostate as we grow older. Finally, an infection in the prostate often causes a rise the PSA blood level.

Digital Exam And Other Indignities

I soon found myself in a small examining room with a young bearded man who asked, "Have you ever had a digital exam?"

At KU Medical Center, only the full doctors got to wear a long white "doctor coat" Medical students were allowed to wear a white jacket that barely went past their waist. Residents had a jacket to mid thigh. Fellows wore somewhat longer coats and the full doctors and professors almost looked like they were wearing a white overcoat. This guy was a resident.

"Is that some kind of computerized exam," I asked. I was that ignorant.

"No."   He smiled. as he put a glove on his hand, lubricated it, and instructed me to drop my pants and bend over. Before I processed what was happening he thrust his large index finger where no man had gone before. So that was the "digit" he was talking about. After feeling around for what seemed like longer than necessary, he withdrew his hand, pulled off his glove and delicately dropped the glove in the trash bin.

I cleaned up, dressed and asked him how things looked (or felt, I guess). Were they Okay?

The resident looked concerned and said the urologist would discuss the results with me. He left the room.

After a lengthy wait, A tall smiling man entered the. room, with the resident and a stern looking Filipino nurse flanking him. He had large hands, and I was glad it was the resident who performed the digital exam.

"Hello, I am Doctor M" he smiled. "Doug here tells me that your digital exam was somewhat irregular. He found a hard lump on your prostate. "

"What does that mean?" I asked.

"It means we ought to look further at your prostate. The digital test only gives part of the information, because it is not possible to feel all parts of the prostate with your finger. Also, your PSA of 4.8 concerns me. Your prostate may be fine, but we need to rule out any possible problems. The next step will be a needle biopsy. "

"OK". I would agree to almost anything at this point. Frankly I was in shock, and my brain was spinning too hard to process much at all. For the second time in an hour, I agreed to a doctor's request without really knowing what was coming next,.

"Good. Say do you have time to do it right now?"

I didn't know enough at the time to know how irregular this request was. I have since learned that prostate biopsies are usually scheduled in advance, prepped with a bowel cleanse and often preceded by preventive antibiotics.

Not this time. I called my wife and gave her the news: I might be running a little late. We were planning to drive from Kansas City to Green Bay Wisconsin to visit her mother in the hospital when I got home from the doctors office. I had fit this appointment in right before we were scheduled to leave.

The Biopsy

The doctor was planning to perform an ultrasound guided needle biopsy of the prostate. This type of biopsy was pretty standard at that time. This procedure is now referred to as a "blind" biopsy, at least by those who believe in the more sophisticated techniques for biopsies that have been developed in recent years, such as an MRI guided biopsy.

I removed my pants and underwear, and pulled on a thin hospital gown, which would soon be lifted right off of my lower half. I then climbed onto a large examining table and assumed the position. I was instructed to lay on my side with my legs drawn up and my posterior exposed.

I couldn't see what was going on, but I could definitely feel it. A large, no, very large rounded ultrasound wand was pushed up my rear, along with a spring loaded needle gun. The doctor looked at a monitor image to aid his aim, and suddenly shot a long hollow needle through the wall of my rectum into my prostate. Even though I was expecting the sample to be taken, the noise of the needle gun and the thrust of the needle made me jump. And it hurt. The needle was pulled out, the sample of prostate tissue removed and the gun loaded with a fresh needle.

This was repeated eight more times. I have read that, at the time this was done, most prostate biopsies were either six or twelve samples. So this doctor evidently split the difference It was somewhat unnerving to hear the doctor and nurse discuss what great samples they were getting.

At last it was over. The doctor cleaned himself up, I cleaned myself up and gave one final urine sample to make sure I didn't have blood in my urine.

I since have had two more prostate biopsies, all at KU. The next two biopsies followed the appropriate procedures including cleansing the colon prior to the test, as well as a preventive course of antibiotics.

My biopsy results didn't seem good compared to other men's results I had read about on line.. Four of my nine samples contained cancer, and they contained a lot of it. The percentages of cancer cells in each sample ranged from 25% to 40%. Parts of my prostate were almost half cancer! And cancer was found on both sides of my prostate.

The good news (or at least better news) was that the samples graded out at a Gleason score 3+3=6.

A Gleason score of six indicated that the cancer was not particularly aggressive or fast growing. The bad news was it was still cancer.

The Gleason score is determined by a pathologist 4looking at samples of the cancer and subjectively deciding how far it varies from normal cells. A Gleason score below six was barely cancer, a score of eight or more was somewhat dire. To complicate things more, I was told that the cells sometimes mutate and can become more aggressive at a later date.

I asked the doctor what he recommended we do. He looked me over and said "How's your heart?"

"Just fine." I answered.

"Good. Then we can schedule you for surgery right away, and get that cancer out of you."

Urologists are surgeons. In fact the Urology Department at KU hospital is called "The Department of Urological Surgery".I had read that Urologists almost always recommended surgery, and Radiation Oncologists almost always recommend radiation. On the other hand, I wanted whichever treatment was right for me.

 "What other options are available?" I asked him.

He mentioned both external radiation and brachytherapy, and offered to refer me to their in house radiation oncologist. He also mentioned cryotherapy, but said they did not do that at KU at that time, but that he could refer me to MD Anderson Cancer Center in Texas if I was interested.

We then discussed side effects of each type of treatment.

What he told me pretty much matched my prior research, but he put a more positive spin on the side effects of surgery. For example, he conceded that surgery had what he said was about a 25% chance of causing impotence, but said "Don't worry, there are plenty of things we can do about that."

I was worried anyway.

He also confirmed the near 100% impotence rate at that time for cryotherapy, which was a relatively new treatment at the time I told him there was no need to look into a referral for that!

We made an appointment with Radiation Oncologist Doctor R.

I then asked how long I could take to make my decision. I had read that in many cases this could be put off for years, although "watchful waiting" was not in vogue yet in 2005. The doctor told me I might have 6 months, based on the amount of cancer I had. He cautioned that I should definitely not wait any longer than that.

I was really too young to be facing this choice. I read that two thirds of all prostate cancer diagnosis were in men over the age of 65. By age 80, 80 per cent of men have some prostate cancer cells. However, prostate cancer diagnosed later in life is usually less aggressive.

But Why me? As part of my research I tried to answer that question.

5 RISK FACTORS FOR PROSTATE CANCER

There are a number of known and suspected risk factors for prostate cancer. It appears a few of them do apply to me.

Age- the older a man is the more likely it is that he has some cancer in his prostate. It is estimated that by age 80 most men will have a slow growing cancer in their prostate. These are the men of whom it can be said "it is more likely they will die with prostate cancer than of it."

Note: I was diagnosed at age 55 so this did not factor into my situation.

Race- Afro-American men are more at risk for prostate cancer and at a younger age. Some guidelines suggest PSA testing for Afro-American men beginning at age 40; other men beginning at age 50.

Note: I am white and still had an early onset at age 55. I knew two men about my age that I worked with and who were diagnosed with prostate cancer about a year before I was. Both are black men who were in shape and ate healthy diets. One even juiced his own organic carrots.

Obesity -It has been shown that us fat guys are more likely to contract prostate cancer than men with a healthy weight.

Note: They got me here. I was 6'3" tall and weighed 380 pounds! I am now 100 pounds lighter. Better late than never.

Diet- There has been a great deal of research associating a high fat red meat diet with prostate cancer. There are also certain foods, such as pomegranate that are considered prostate healthy.

Note: They got me again. I was definitely a meat and potatoes kind of guy.

Family history. - Men who have close relatives who have had prostate cancer are at higher risk themselves of developing cancer.

Note: I am not aware of any relatives of mine who had prostate cancer

Genetic factors- recent research indicates that certain gene defects can make a man more likely to develop prostate cancer.

Risk factors are not destiny. They do not explain every case of prostate cancer. But if it is not too late for you, I would pay attention. I was certainly ignorant.

6 COMPARING BRACHYTHERAPY AND SURGERY

Talking with Other Patients and Comparing Treatments

Two men I worked with had been treated for prostate cancer the year before. One chose seed therapy, the other opted for surgery. I talked to them both. The man who had surgery told me about his decision making process. His wife had strongly told him "Get that cancer out of you before it has a chance to spread!" Decision made.

I could see some logic in that. Once the cancer has metastasized (spread) outside the prostate it cannot be cured. Treatments are given to slow its growth as long as possible.

. According to Memorial Sloan Kettering hospital, one of the premier treatment centers in the country, pretty much every patient is incontinent immediately after prostate removal. Eventually about 90 per cent of them regain control, which of course means 10 per cent of them never do.

In contrast, Web MD indicates that urinary incontinence from brachytherapy is rare. Some men experience a burning when urinating and some have a hard time emptying their bladder. Both conditions are normally controlled with medication.

Memorial Sloan Kettering hospital also indicated that every prostate surgery patient will be impotent immediately after surgery. Often it is not possible to spare the nerves that enable erections due to the exact nature and extent of the cancer. Most doctors do not like to give percentages of the number of men who regain erections. Most commonly, studies indicate that the number who become sexually functional may be 50 to 75 percent, but only with Viagra or other medications. It is not unusual for men to resort to a vacuum pump, shots in the penis, or even a penile implant to make the penis artificially stiff.

With seed therapy, impotence is not usually an immediate problem. Problems are more likely to occur which patients are a number of years out, but virtually all men experience more problems

Radiation patients do sometimes have bowel symptoms that surgery patients do not. These may include increased frequency, occasional bowel leakage or bleeding. These are not common and often get better after the seeds have used up their radioactivity.

The following chart compares the two options I was considering. Adding hormone therapy to either of them would complicate matters

Side Effect	Prostatectomy surgery	Brachytherapy seeds
Urinary incontinence	100% to begin with, still 10% after one year.	Not to begin with. Some incontinence may begin after several years
Impotence	100% to begin with. May still be 50% ongoing. May need pills, pumps or penile implant	Not initially. Some ED may start after several years. It usually responds well to pills such as Viagra or Cialis.
Bowel symptoms	Not Usually	Less than 10% of patients have increased bowel frequency or even leakage

Catheter usage	100% need a catheter the first few weeks at home. Occasional patients need one ongoing.	Seeds are usually implanted outpatient and patients go home without a catheter.
Penile Shrinkage	Anecdotally, yes It could be that shortening the ureter pulls the penis further back into the body.	No.

7 RADIATION ONCOLOGY CONSULT AND PREPARATION FOR SEED INSERTION

"Radiation oncology" is a scary name for a department. The sign in bold letters on the front of the squat building "Radiation Oncology "shouted at me " You have cancer. ". And I felt like everyone seeing me walk into that building knew I had cancer.

Once inside, my wife and I took the elevator to the underground check in. The entire office with its heavy equipment and potentially dangerous radiation was entirely underground. I learned that this was a common arrangement in most radiation treatment centers.

We soon ended up in a room with the Radiation

Oncologist's resident assistant. He read my chart and discussed the differences between exterior beam radiation therapy(EBRT) and brachytherapy, or seeds. However,, he said, I was not a candidate for exterior radiation because of my size. There was just too much excess flesh for the radiation to penetrate through on the way to the prostate and too great a chance for collateral damage. I might be a candidate for seeds though. It would depend on how prostate imaging turned out, assuming I chose that course.

In LDR or low dose brachytherapy, tiny rice sized pellets of titanium filled with a radioactive agent are inserted directly into the prostate. The number and placement of the seeds is dependent on the size of the prostate. The intent is to kill the cancer cells while avoiding damage to the surrounding tissue. The radiation in the seeds is depleted in six months or so, but the seeds remain permanently in the prostate.

There is another procedure called HDR or high dose radiation brachytherapy, in which higher doses of radiation are delivered directly into the prostate via wires or tubes, and then withdrawn. This is a newer procedure and was not offered to me in 2005.

I asked how many seed procedures Dr R performed. I had read that a key to success in either surgery or seeds was to select a doctor with a lot of experience, performing at least 5 to 10 procedures per month.

"Last year he did 12 ".

"Only one per month? "I was concerned.

He explained that the Urologists seldom referred anyone for a Radiation consultation, instead talking practically everyone into surgery

He did leave us with a little ditty minimizing my concern about my incontinence. Everyone eventually has some issues with it eventually

"It doesn't matter how much you shake or how much you dance, the last few drops always go in your pants. "

We were more embarrassed than amused.

We were then joined by Dr. R He was a small oriental man with a spark in his eye who seemed excited to have a referral from Urology. He repeated much of what the resident had said. He was enthusiastic about performing brachytherapy on me. We went ahead to make an appointment for imaging and measuring to see if I was a candidate for seed therapy.

A week later I was in a basement room preparing to have my prostate measured. This, in combination with an MRI and X-Ray would determine if I was physiologically a good candidate for the process. Some men's prostates were too big compared to their pelvic bones, and it was not possible for the needles to reach all needed areas of the prostate.

Prostate Mapping Attempt

I was placed on an operating room table, on my back with my legs in stirrups, my privates and rear end fully exposed to the room and exposed to the nurse that prepped me. I was getting used to this indignity. It had become obvious that any shred of modesty disappeared when prostate problems arise.

Suddenly I noticed that there was a floor to ceiling plate glass window with no curtains in the wall directly opposite my feet. This offered a full view of what i didn't really want anyone to see.

When the resident entered to perform the prostate measuring I asked him if anyone ever walked by that window. He laughed.

"That is a window well. We are twelve feet underground and no one can peek in. "

I was glad to hear that.

The resident then proceeded to insert a large medical instrument up my rear. Unfortunately, I was getting used to this, and endured without too much pain. However as he twisted the instrument within me, he abruptly stopped, with a distressed look on his face and told me we were done.

After I got dressed Dr. R joined us and told me that they had been unable to complete the measurement. I believe it had something to do with my size.

Without really explaining why, Dr. R said he wanted to refer me to a Dr. John Sheldon at Research hospital. "He has better equipment and does a lot more of these procedures."

I then waited while he called the other doctor and told him he was referring me. The only explanation i heard was "He is really big!"

Fate had blessed me with the right doctor. Sometimes morbid obesity has its benefits

A week later, I repeated the prostate mapping procedure at another hospital across town. This was a totally different experience.

The table for my prostate measuring at Research Hospital was not underground and the room did not have windows. My privacy was assured, except for the 4 or 5 people observing my nether regions. I was arranged on a table by a couple of nurses. I was in a slightly awkward position with my uncovered rear end poking into the air. Then the anesthesiologist put a mask on me and i was out. I woke up in the recovery room and heard that everything had gone well.

The average prostate is 15 to 30 cubic centimeters (cc). My prostate clocked in at about 65 cc. Many patients with this large of a prostate are either told that they do not qualify for brachytherapy seeds, or are placed on hormone therapy for several months, in order to shrink the prostate. Fortunately wide pelvises run in my family, so I was still able to have prostate seeds. There was plenty of room between my pelvic bones to get the needles in.

The Seed Insertion Process

The measurements from the prostate mapping, along with a collection of x rays, CT scans, and MRI's are fed into a computer that determines the exact number of titanium seeds filled with Iodine-125 are needed and plots the precise best placement of the seeds. They are placed in a pattern that should irradiate the prostate completely but spare surrounding tissues from damage.

The next step is the seed insertion procedure itself.

It was determined that I would have 76 I-125 seeds inserted. First I would have the ultrasound wand once more into my rectum. Thankfully this time I will be asleep. This needed to follow very shortly after the imaging to ensure there are no changes in the prostate position or size prior to the procedure. Seventy six long needles each with a seed on the end would be Inserted through the perineum (between the scrotum and the anus) into the prostate. No actual incision is needed. The flesh was supposed to close back up after the needles were withdrawn. No stitches or even band aids would be needed.

The entire procedure normally takes about 90 minutes. If all goes well it will be an outpatient procedure and I will go home the same day. In contrast to prostatectomy patients, seed patients go home Without A CATHETER!

8 MY OPERATION AND TYPICAL RESULTS

The following Monday I was prepped and on the operating table by 8 am. I went to sleep with the help of some nice drugs and woke up a few hours later in the recovery room, By the feel of it, I wasn't sure if 76 needles or 76 trombones had been shoved through my perineum. I woke up with a catheter, but it was taken out not long after I came to.

I wasn't awake to see it, but I was told that a custom molded piece of equipment held the needles in the perfect computer proscribed distance. from each other. The ultrasound wand was used to view that each was placed in the correct depth.

The doctor came in to see me after I had my wits about me. Things went well, he said. i could leave as soon as I could urinate.

By four o'clock in the afternoon, I still had not urinated. The doctor checked on me again and said he was confident I could go home anyway and things would start flowing when I was free of performance anxiety.

My wife drove me home slowly and carefully, and put me to bed. She did not lay as close as usual to me out of concern for both of us.

The Iodine-125 seeds have a half life of 60 days and deliver the major part of their radiation in that period. However the seeds keep releasing radiation for about six months. I was instructed not to hold children on my lap and to stay at least 3 feet away from pregnant women for the first several months.

The effect of the radiation on the body is cumulative. The radiation slowly destroys the cancer cells within a few millimeters of each seed. By the end of six months all cancer cells will be permanently damaged and will gradually die off rather than reproducing. This assumes that the seed placement was correct.

Healthy prostate cells. actually tolerate the radiation better than cancer cells and many of them survive and still function. Because of this, seed patients still have PSA. This PSA drops rapidly over the first few months, and then continues to drop as more cancer cells die off, and as more healthy cells live but become scar tissue.

Using PSA To Monitor Success

PSA provides a more accurate measure of treatment success than it does of initially finding prostate cancer. Because the prostate is either removed or radiated, most PSA being produced in the years after initial treatment are almost curtaining being produced by rogue cancer cells which escaped the initial treatment. Usually, they were already outside the prostate prior to initial diagnosis, even if not detected until later.

If a surgery patient's operation is successful, their PSA drops down to zero.. Any reappearance of PSA, even in very small amounts, indicates that the cancer may have spread elsewhere in the body before surgery was performed.

In contrast, a seed patient's PSA gradually drops over about a two year period. It does not go to zero, because seed patients still have some healthy prostate tissue. The low point reached in each person's PSA is called the nadir, and PSA typically will continue to fluctuate close to that level. However, If the PSA rises two points above that nadir, a recurrence of cancer is suspected.

42

9.THE AFTERMATH

I felt pretty good the first few weeks after the seeds were put in. I was a little tender in the perineum. As the low dose of radiation continued to fry my prostate tissue, sitting down became more painful. The American Brachytherapy Society indicates that most Brachytherapy patients are able to regain normal activity 3 to 4 days after the procedure. This was my experience too, and I returned to work about a week after receiving the seeds.

The biggest challenge I had to start with was keeping my dog' head out of my lap! Theodora was a 60 pound lap dog. Tan, she was part Labrador and part Husky. Theodora was a nurturing dog, with a talent for resting her head whenever a person is hurting. She insisted on resting her head immediately over my prostate any time I sat or laid down. She was extremely strong, perhaps due to the husky in her, and could not be moved easily if she did not want to be moved. I was unable to do a good job of shielding her from the radiation.

There have been studies reporting that dogs are able to detect cancer in people. Several Web Md articles and other sources have indicated that dogs have detected colon cancer by sniffing stool samples or breath and lung cancer by sniffing breath samples A PBS News hour story from Sept 6 2014 indicated that some researchers believe dogs can detect prostate cancer by sniffing urine samples. That said, it is unlikely the "dog scan" will ever replace the cat scan. But in some circles it may become an additional non-invasive all natural test.

My Side effects of seed therapy.

By about the third week though, the radiation effects on my body were building. I started feeling more and more fatigue. I also felt, not pain, but a fullness and feeling of discomfort in my prostate area. Prior to receiving the seeds, I could not really sense where my prostate was in my body. Now it was obvious.

I didn't have the rectal bleeding a small number of patients have, but I did find that a large bowel movement put uncomfortable pressure on my prostate Some people find stool softeners helpful to alleviate this symptom..this symptom..

I did not have urinary leakage. On the contrary, I had been prescribed Flo-max in order to be able to urinate. Typically seed patients have urinary urgency but difficulty emptying the bladder. Medication can help with this condition and is usually prescribed initially and decreased to zero over the first year.

We have been discussing the other bodily functions, so i guess we need to talk about sex. After seed therapy sex can normally be resumes when the discomfort in the perineum (where the seeds were inserted) has subsided.

Many references recommend using a condom for the first few months. The semen is often bloody or discolored (gross!) and it is possible though unlikely that a radioactive seed may escape in the semen. As the radiation continues to turn more and more of the prostate into scar tissue, the volume of semen will decrease.

I am not going to share all of my personal details in this area, except to say everything still worked. This vindicated my choice of treatment. I did have some difficulties occur about 3 years into treatment, which I will discuss later.

10 MY PSA TRACKING AFTER BRACYTHERAPY

In the three months following the seed insertion, I did have very mild urinary leakage, and my libido was dampened by the radiation. I was able to perform. My biggest surprise was the fatigue I started to experience.

My PSA progress was good. My first PSA after the procedure was 1.56, down from a high of 5.3. I was concerned that it was not descending quickly enough.

Brachytherapy patients typically alternate appointments with their radiology oncologist (rad onc) and their urologist. This process was complicated in my case, because my rad onc and my urologist practiced at different hospitals. I wasn't really sure how often they communicated together, and sometimes thought I was receiving contradictory instructions.

I had an appointment with the Urologist Dr M at the three month mark in January 2006. He performed the dreaded DRE (Digital Rectal Exam) and proclaimed it good. The radiation had shrunk my prostate so much that he couldn't feel it. He also said he was very pleased with the drop in my PSA. He also noted that imaging of my prostate showed the seeds placement looks good

My PSAs continued to trend downward, which was a sign that the cancer cells continued to die off. I was retested every three months, with the following results.

12/29/2005 1.56 PSA

4/3/2006 0.79 PSA

07/03/2006 0.68 PSA

11/01/2006 0.57 PSA

01/08/2007 0.54 PSA

03/05/2007 1.01 PSA?????

Why did that go up? Was the cancer back?

PSA Bounce

Oops! Now that was concerning. I talked to my oncologist about this and he assured me that I was experiencing the scary PSA bounce. This is common in brachytherapy patients. About 50 per cent of brachytherapy patients experience an upward bounce in their PSA. Assuming the PSA resumes its downward journey, this is nothing to be concerned about.

A CBS News/Web MD article from November 6, 2006 discusses a study which indicated that the ten year survival rate for brachytherapy patients who experienced a bounce was actually 4 per cent higher than those patients who did not experience a bounce. About 33 to 50 per cent of seed patients have an upward bounce in their PSA.

I did not discover any research that definitively explained why some patients have a bounce and some don't. One theory that makes sense, and which I like, is that the PSA bounces because a large number of cancer cells died and released their PSA into bloodstream. DIE CANCER DIE!

Radiation damages cancer cells but does not always kill them immediately. The cancer cells are incapacitated and cannot reproduce. When they finally pass away they release their debris into the bloodstream. thus raising the PSA.

Fortunately, my PSA resumed its downward trajectory.

04/09/2007. 0.52 PSA

07/13/2007. 0.51 PSA

11/04/2007. 0.47 PSA

The Prostate Strikes Back

On May 11 2008, my prostate counterattacked me. It had apparently taken all the abuse it cared to, and was determined to speak out about it, using all the tools at its disposal.

 First, I noticed blood in my urine. Second, I had a shooting pain in my prostate. Third, I literally could not pee. No urination, nothing I did have uncomfortable pressure building in my bladder, with no way to relieve it.

This seemed like an emergency to me

I called the radiation doctor first. He told me this was a case for the urologist. I only hoped urology would not pass me back to him. Fortunately, Urology was able to give me a same day appointment. I didn't want just any emergency room doctor poking around down there.

 I arrived at the hospital and was ushered

immediately into an examining room where a nurse performed an ultrasound of my bladder. She confirmed that, yes, I did need to urinate, and no I had not exploded yet. I was getting less comfortable by the minute.

A resident physician came in, listened to my sad story and opined that I would have to go home and self catheter until such time as the doctor could treat me.

 I prayed he was wrong. I needed immediate relief!

The resident was wrong. Doctor H said he had time and said he would perform a cystoscopy to find out what was going on. In a cystoscopy a very small camera with a light is run up the penis through the prostate, all the way to the bladder.

I soon found myself in a gown on a table with stirrups with my nether regions exposed once again. A nurse joined me in the room with me to prep me for the procedure.

She proceeded to squirt a tube of numbing gel into the tip of my penis and slowly massaged it all the way up to my pelvis. This was definitely the least erotic penis massage I had ever had!

Dr. H then entered the room. He put on a pair of goggles with a long thin wire protruding from it. It kind of looked like a World War One gas mask with an anteater feature added.

He proceeded to feed the other end of the flexible tube up my penis, which was definitely NOT entirely numb. The good doctor kept up a running commentary of what he was seeing as he slowly fed the camera further and further into me.

When the camera got to the prostate Dr. H said he was pleased to see I did not have a blockage. What I did have was a raw spot on the inside of the ureter where it was passing through the prostate. He explained that every time urine hit that spot my prostate would spasm, cutting off the flow. He then extended the camera all the way to my bladder and looked around to be sure that the bladder was not the source of bleeding, and to do a visual check for bladder cancer. Fortunately everything checked out OK there.

After he pulled the camera back out (what relief) and I was dressed, he gave me two prescriptions which effectively soothed my prostate. They did turn my urine orange, but that just reminded me they were working. My plumbing resumed working, so the self catheter process was avoided.

Unfortunately, mild bleeding and pain reoccurred

later that year. The urologist performed a repeat biopsy just to be sure nothing ominous was happening. Nothing was. Finally, in November 2008 my rad onc prescribed a combination of Avodart and ibuprofen which resolved the irritation and bleeding in my prostate.

I Go On A Mild Form Of Hormone Therapy

The Avodart (generic dutesteride), had three major effects, two good and one bad.

On the good side, the Avodart resolved the inflammation in my prostate. As a second bonus, it stimulated hair growth. Aside from its primary purposes, avodart stimulates hair growth, much like Romaine.

On the major bad side, the Avodart pretty much wiped out my libido. Whether I could perform sexually or not, it seldom occurred to me to try.

Avodart is primarily prescribed for men with BPH, or enlarged prostate. Its primary effect is to shrink the prostate. It is a hormone blocking drug, but unlike Lupron and other commonly prescribed anti-androgen drugs, Avodart does not block the production of testosterone. Instead, it blocks the conversion of testosterone to DHT, a more potent form of the male hormone. One result of this treatment is that the prostate shrinks. Which is why it works so well for enlarged prostate.

In addition to resolving my painful urination problems, the change in medication put my PSA back on a downward track. Eventually, it reached a nadir (low point) of 0.17 and fluctuated around that level for several years.

At the five years after treatment mark in October 2010, my PSA was 0.5 and I was declared cancer free.

Chance Of Recurrence

Even when declared cured, we cancer patients are always looking over our shoulders to see if a cancer recurrence is sneaking up on us. Every ache or pain concerns us. Did a few rogue cells escape before the original tumor was removed or radiated? This is referred to as micro-metastases. No matter how good things looked after the original treatment, there are no guarantees.

My book <u>When Cancer Escapes the Prostate</u> explores what happens if things go wrongl.

10. Additional Resources

The science of treating prostate cancer has dramatically improved in the twelve years since I was diagnosed. There are a number of new tests available that give a better picture of the location and severity of the cancer. MRI guided biopsies and more sophisticated whole body scans are examples.

There have been a number of new treatments developed, some with enticing names such as Cyberknife and Proton Beam.

There has been an explosion in the understanding and use of Active Surveillance (AS). Many men are postponing treatment and its side effects until absolutely necessary.

Researching prostate cancer information and options can be quite confusing. For comprehensive and up to date information consider the following sources.

US TOO International

i recommend Us Too International at
http://www.ustoo.org/

A number of excellent discussion forums which

can be linked through their website. There are enough men (and women) in the forums that there is always someone who has had a similar experience to you and can share their story, advice and support. Topics include

Newly diagnosed

Treatment Options

Active Surveillance

Managing side effects

Exercise and Nutrition

Wives, Families, Friends and Caregivers

Prostate Cancer and Intimacy

Screening and Early Detection

Recurrence/Advanced Disease

Clinical Trials

In addition, Us Too sponsors local support groups in many metropolitan areas.

Finally, Us Too offers a large number of free written resources for prostate cancer patients.

I am referring readers to this group because they are my number one go to source for information of any kind of information and support concerning prostate cancer.. I participate in their online forums, have received excellent written material from them, and receive a daily Us Too email.

Live Strong

When I was first diagnosed, I received a great deal of excellent information from the Live Strong organization.. They provide a plethora of resources for patients with any type of cancer, not just prostate cancer. I received a free binder from them designed to keep track of all the test results and other information I received from the doctors. I heartily recommend them. They can be reached at https://livestrong.org/

You Are Not Alone Now

YANA _ You are Not Alone Now is a patient run prostate cancer support site, based in Australia. Their web site contains extensive resources for the newly diagnosed patient. My favorite feature is a unique chart listing hundreds of prostate cancer patients' diagnostic information, type of treatment chosen, and results of treatment. The chart also tracks their progress over the years, including side effects and any recurrence. Entries are made by the patients or their families and contain valuable anecdotal information They can be reached at http://www.yananow.org/

Thank You

Thank you for the opportunity to share my prostate journey with you. I pray that my story has been helpful and educational for you..

About the Author

59

Lonnie Boyd is a 13 year prostate cancer survivor. He is a veteran of the prostate wars.

Mr. Boyd is retired after 34 years as a regional official of the United States Social Security Administration. He is involved in ministry to people with Special Needs, especially those on the autistic spectrum.

Other Books by Lonnie Boyd

Lonnie Boyd is also the author of the following books, They are available both as e-books and in paperback.

When Cancer Escapes The Prostate: Treatments For Advanced Prostate Cancer

Prostate cancer that is contained in the prostate can be successfully eradicated by any of several initial treatments.
But when prostate cancer spreads outside the prostate, the treatment options change. Rather than seeking a cure, patients and doctors try to delay the growth of cancer while considering the effects of various treatments on quality of life.

Talking To God About Cancer: Prayers For Patients And Their Loved Ones

A cancer diagnosis for yourself or a loved one stirs

up thoughts and concerns that can stun and overwhelm. This book provides prayer starters, scriptures and reflections to help the reader find peace, comfort and strength when facing the challenge of cancer.

www.ingramcontent.com/pod-product-compliance
Lightning Source LLC
Chambersburg PA
CBHW060208260726

48658CB00005BA/1944